The 5:2 Diet

The Simple Way to Burn Fat & Stay Lean for Life

Thomas Rohmer

Table of Contents

Introduction:

Every year, millions of people go on a diet with the hopes of losing weight and getting in shape. Sadly, most of these people will not be successful—and it makes sense as to why. Most diets set you up to fail right from the start.

They'll restrict your favorite foods and cut your calories down to dangerously low levels all for the sake of fast results. The problem is that even if you do lose some weight with these extreme methods, you won't be able to sustain it for life. You'll quit when you can't take it anymore, and that's when rebound weight gain will start to occur.

Fortunately the 5:2 diet is far different from your typical diet. It's a simple and easy approach to fat loss that you can do for a long time to come. You'll not only be able to lose the weight in the first place, but keep it off—for good. If that sounds good to you, then you're in the right place.

In this book, you'll learn all of the ins and outs of the 5:2 diet. You'll also be given low calorie and high protein recipes to help you execute on the diet, and I've even included a workout routine you can do. Yes, this book is about the 5:2 diet, but I want to give you all of the tools you'll need to be successful with fitness. Let's get started...

Chapter 1: Why the 5:2 Diet is Different

Why is it that every year so many people struggle to lose weight and successfully keep it off? The reason is because most diets set you up to fail right from the get go. Tell me if this has ever happened to you:

1. You want to lose weight.
2. You go on a diet.
3. You eliminate all junk food and eat healthy 24/7.
4. After a week, you start to get worn out.
5. You get tempted by a chocolate chip cookie and eat it.
6. You feel guilty and binge eat everything in sight.
7. A few days later, when you're feeling better about yourself, you start the process over again.

Was it your fault if something similar to this has happened to you before? Definitely not. Many diets sound good on paper, but they're hard to live by. As humans, we have desires to eat sugary and salty foods, and that's completely okay when eaten in the right amounts.

We're not robots that can be programmed to eat salads for the rest of our lives. We need practicality in our nutrition plans, and unfortunately most diets treat us like we're robots! That's why in order to see lasting results, you must do something different from the norm. And luckily, the 5:2 diet is different from your average weight loss diet.

What Makes the 5:2 Diet Different?

The key difference between the 5:2 diet and most other weight loss diets is the fact that the 5:2 diet is sustainable for a long period of time. Normally, you'll be busting your butt going through hunger pangs and cravings in order to make a noticeable difference in how you look. Unfortunately though, you have nothing to look forward to except for more pain and misery. This gets to be demotivating after awhile no matter how good the results are, and you'll eventually quit.

It's as if you have to choose between living a normal live and not being satisfied with your fitness level, or be happy with how you look, but be miserable with the process of getting and staying fit. Conversely, with the 5:2 diet, you'll be able to get in shape in a very non-intrusive manner. Most of the time you'll be eating how you normally do, which is great if you want to fly under the radar and not tell everyone you know you're going on a diet.

Of course, some changes will still have to be made—you can't keep everything the same and start hoping for changes to magically happen. However, the changes you'll have to make will be easy to fit in with your lifestyle no matter how busy you are. This is what'll allow you to continue doing the 5:2 diet for a long time to come. You see, whatever you initially did to lose weight, you must keep doing to keep the weight off. If you revert back to your old ways, you'll slowly start to gain all of the weight back.

Most nutrition plans are good at helping you lose 20 plus pounds in a few short weeks. The problem is that they leave you stranded for what to do after that initial weight is lost. How are you supposed to keep it off? With the 5:2 diet, you'll be able to make a smooth transition between losing weight and maintaining your new goal bodyweight once you reach it. Yes, this is a book about the 5:2 "diet", but I don't like thinking of it as a diet. The word diet implies short-term change. If you go on a diet, you must eventually come off of that diet, and that's when rebound weight gain will typically occur. On the other hand, the 5:2 diet is a lifestyle nutrition plan. It's something that you'll easily be able to do and see success with for the rest of your life.

Chapter 2: The Caloric Deficit is King, Not Your Diet

Many people think that the only way you lose weight is by going on a diet and eating healthy foods. Most people have no idea how your body actually works in regards to burning fat. As you'll soon find out, calories matter way more than the diet you're following.

The diet is simply the means by which you'll be reducing your caloric intake. For example, if you go on a low-carb diet, you won't be guaranteed to lose weight even if you're following it correctly. Something else must be in place, but before I get into that, it's first important to understand exactly what a calorie is.

What Exactly is a Calorie Anyway?

You've undoubtedly heard of the word calorie before. But what exactly is a calorie anyway? Is it something evil you should avoid whenever possible? Is it the bane of your existence?

Many people have an idea of what a calorie is, but most don't know. If you went out on the street and asked 10 different people what a calorie is, you'd likely get 10 different answers. Here's the textbook definition of a calorie:

"The energy needed to raise the temperature of 1 gram of water through 1° C"

Sounds complicated right? Essentially, a calorie is a measurement of energy. Your body is constantly undergoing chemical reactions to keep you alive. All of these chemical reactions (digestion, breathing, organ function, etc.) require energy.

Your body gets the energy necessary to continue functioning from the food (calories) you eat. Calories aren't your worst enemy; they're your friend. You have to work with them, not against them. And as you're about to find out, not all calories are the same.

Why the Caloric Deficit is King

Pop quiz: What's the *only* way your body can burn fat?

If you looked at the title above and guessed caloric deficit, then you'd be correct! A caloric deficit is simply when you burn off more calories than you consume. The opposite is a caloric surplus—consuming more calories than you burn off. And maintenance is when you are at a caloric equilibrium.

Here's an example:

- Joe burns 2,000 calories a day and eats 1,800. He's in a caloric deficit of 200 calories and he'll start to lose weight.
- Joe burns 2,000 calories a day and eats 2,200. He's in a caloric surplus of 200 calories and he'll start to gain weight.
- Joe burns 2,000 calories a day and eats 2,000. He's at maintenance and will not gain or lose weight.

As I mentioned earlier, every day your body needs energy (calories) in order to continue on with all of its chemical functions such as breathing, digesting food, organ function, etc. The amount of calories you burn in any given day is your resting metabolic rate (rmr). Once you figure out your body's rmr, you can then determine how many calories you need to eat to start burning fat.

Determining your rmr is simple—multiply your bodyweight in pounds by 13.
Let's use myself as an example:

Bodyweight=195 pounds
195 x 13= RMR of 2,535

This means that if I eat less than 2,535 calories I'll be in a caloric deficit and I'll start to lose weight. If I eat more than 2,535 calories I'll be in a caloric surplus and I'll start to gain weight. And finally, if I eat exactly 2,535 calories, I'll be at maintenance and I'll neither gain nor lose weight.

The question is—how big of a caloric deficit do you need to create in order for it to translate into pounds lost? There's about 3,500 calories in one pound of fat (1), meaning that you must create a cumulative caloric deficit of 3,500 calories in order to lose 1 pound. So if you divide 3,500 by 7 days in a week, you'll need to create an average daily caloric deficit of 500 calories to lose 1 pound per week.

Referring back to the example from above, here's what that would translate to:

RMR- 2,535 − 500= 2,035

This means that I need to eat 2,035 calories everyday if I want to lose 1 pound per week. The more weight you have to lose, the larger the caloric deficit you can create. For example, you could eat at a caloric deficit of 750 calories and lose 1.5 pounds per week, or you could eat at a deficit of 1,000 calories to lose 2 pounds per week.

Essentially, for every 250 calories you can expect to lose an additional .5-pound. The key is to not get carried away. You might want to lose all of the weight as soon as possible and jump right into a 1,000-calorie caloric deficit.

That may not be the best idea. For most people, losing 1 pound per week by creating a 500-calorie caloric deficit is golden. Imagine yourself a year from now being 52 pounds lighter without having to put forth much effort! That's much better than spinning your wheels trying to lose 100 pounds in that same time frame.

Here's how you can determine the rate you should lose weight at:

- If you need to lose between 5-10 pounds, then aim for .5 pound of weight loss per week.
- If you need to lose between 10-30 pounds, then aim for 1 pound of weight loss per week.
- If you need to lose 30+ pounds, then aim for 1.5-2+ pounds of weight loss per week.

What if you don't know how much weight you need to lose to look the way you want to? This is a good question because you won't know how much you need to weigh to look good until you reach that point. Therefore, you'll simply have to take your best guess as to what your goal weight is and adjust it once you reach it.

For example, let's say someone weighs 200 pounds. This individual could pick a goal weight of 180 pounds and start losing weight at a rate of 1 pound per week. Once he reaches his goal of 180 pounds, he can see if he's satisfied with how he looks.

If he's happy with how he looks, then great. If not, then he needs to readjust his goal. He could set his new target weight at 170 pounds and lose weight at a rate of .5 to 1 pound per week, continuing the process until he's happy with his leanness.

Chapter 3: History and Benefits of Fasting

The 5:2 diet is a type of fasting diet. Before I get into the specific ins and outs of the diet, it's first important to understand the history behind fasting and some of the many benefits it can provide you with. Fasting isn't a new idea, even though it has gained popularity in recent times. People have been fasting for thousands of years for various reasons—religious purposes, preparing for war, political protests, healing of illnesses (before medicine became prevalent), and even out of necessity. Muslims fast while the sun is up during the month of Ramadan.

Roman Catholics fast for 40 days during Lent to represent the 40 days Jesus fasted in the desert. Judaism has several annual fasts as well. Fasting was sometimes demanded before going to war as part of a ritual. And figures like Mahatma Gandhi have fasted for 21 days straight during the struggle for Indian independence.

It wasn't until recently that people began fasting for the enhanced health and fat loss benefits. Imagine for a second that you're a nomadic hunter and gather living thousands of years ago. Every day when you wake up, you can't simply go to the fridge and get something to eat. You must earn your food for the day by hunting for it.

Therefore, a lot of hunters had to fast because there wasn't anything to eat in the morning. Fast-forward to the present day and things are much different. Today, there's an overabundance of food. Anytime you want, you can drive through a 24/7 fast food restaurant and get something to eat.

You don't have to burn calories hunting for your food; you get in your car and drive to go get it. This is part of the reason why there is an obesity epidemic in America. Yes, having convenient restaurants and grocery stores is awesome, but they come at a price.

We're no longer forced to delay eating or have to earn it with exercise. How many people tell themselves, "I'll only eat this burger if I exercise for 30 minutes," or, "I'll eat this burger for lunch, but I won't eat anything else until then so I don't overeat." No one does this! It's easier to eat the burger now and worry about the consequences later.

Are We Even Meant to Eat Breakfast Anyway?

You've undoubtedly heard things before like, "Breakfast is the most important meal of the day," or, "Start your day off right with a good balanced breakfast." But were we even meant to eat breakfast anyway? Our ancestors didn't eat breakfast.

 They had to wake up and hunt for their food. They didn't have an endless amount of cereal and pastries at their fingertips right when they woke up. So what happened? It wasn't until the 15th century that the word breakfast came into use in written English to describe a morning meal.

So the idea of breakfast has been around for quite some time, but it wasn't until recently that it became popularized. It all started with two men, Will Keith Kellogg and C.W. Post, creating their own cereal companies—Kellogg Company and Postum Cereal Company (now known as Post Cereals). The key to these companies' success came down to two factors— sugar and marketing.

Thanks to a barrage of advertising, cereal was able to maintain a reputation that it was a healthy food. It would even go as far as to claim that cereal cured everything up to malaria and appendicitis. This was even the start of claims such as, "a good source of Vitamin D!"

And to appeal to children, companies created cartoon mascots such as Tony the Tiger and Snap, Crackle, and Pop, which started appearing around the 1930s. Finally, there's the phrase, "breakfast is the most important meal of the day." Cereal companies must first convince you to eat breakfast, and then get you to buy their cereal.

If they can do that, then they're in the clear because most people eat the same thing for breakfast everyday. Additionally, cereal was fast and convenient to make, which became increasingly important as corporate America was developing in the industrial age. Breakfast is a meal just like lunch or dinner. And while it may not be the most important, it certainly is the most marketed meal of the three.

Benefits of Fasting

Aside from making fat loss a breeze, what else can you expect to gain from a fasting nutrition plan like the 5:2 diet? Quite a few things as it turns out...

-Live a longer life: There is evidence to suggest that fasting can help improve lifespan (2).

-Your body will become more efficient at using fat for fuel (3): When you fast, your body becomes glycogen depleted. Your body will then use fat stores for energy, and therefore learn to use fat for fuel for more effectively.

-Fasting can help to improve cognitive brain function, which will help to improve learning (4).

-Increased human growth hormone levels (hgh) (5): HGH is an important hormone for developing a lean and muscular body. It's responsible for muscle and bone growth, regulation of fluids, and regulation of body composition.

-You'll save time and money: Think about it. You won't have to spend as much time preparing, cooking, and eating meals. Plus, you'll save money at the grocery store!

-Improve focus and concentration: Have you ever felt sluggish or sleepy after eating a meal? The reason is because carbs make tryptophan more accessible to the brain. The tryptophan gets converted into serotonin, which eventually turns into melatonin. Melatonin regulates sleep and increases drowsiness. Therefore, by skipping breakfast you'll be more alert and focused, allowing you to be more productive in the morning.

-Faster recovery from sickness: There is evidence to suggest that fasting can help the body save energy and reduce heat loss, thus allowing it to focus solely on fighting off infection (6).

-Fasting may have positive effects on insulin resistance, thus reducing risk for type 2 diabetes (7).

-Fasting can help to reduce total cholesterol, blood pressure, and triglycerides (8).

Chapter 4: What is the 5:2 Diet?

The 5:2 diet is a method of intermittent fasting that was popularized by Michael Mosley. Essentially, during five days of the week you'll eat as you normally would. Then on the other two days, you'll fast and consume 2-3 small meals for a total of roughly 500 calories for women and 600 for men.

The 5:2 diet is more of a pattern of eating than a typical diet. This is because most of the time you'll be eating how you usually do, and you'll only be making changes two days of the week. That's much different from a normal diet where you'll be making drastic changes to your eating habits seven days of the week.

Not only that, but the 5:2 diet is very flexible. You're only being asked to make dietary changes two days of the week, which makes it easy to fit in with your schedule. If you're on a standard diet, what will you do when an event such as a wedding comes up? Will you make an exception and cheat on your nutritional plan? Or will you be "that guy" who's too good to eat any of the delicious food provided and bring brown rice in a Tupperware dish?

The 5:2 diet allows you to pick which two days you want to fast on. So whenever something like a wedding is coming up, you can simply plan accordingly. The only rule to this is that there must be at least one non-fasting day in between your fasting days. Having back-to-back fasting days would be far too drastic and unnecessary.

Usually you'll want to plan to have your fasting days on the days when you're the busiest. Don't fast on a Saturday for example if you know that you're likely going to eat at a restaurant with your family. Instead, plan them on busy workdays when you have a bunch of meetings or your kids are busy with extracurricular activities. You'll want to keep yourself distracted because cutting your calories so low on fasting days can be difficult to get used to at first.

It's also important to note that you're not given a free pass to eat whatever you want whenever you want on your five normal days of eating. Ideally you want to eat the same amount of food as if you hadn't been fasting at all. If a day of normal eating for you consists of regularly binge eating on junk, then maybe it's time to change your definition of normal.

You're not immune to calories because you're fasting two days out of the week. The laws of thermodynamics and calorie balance still apply to you, which means that it could be possible for you to still gain weight while on the 5:2 diet simply because you're over consuming calories on the five regular days of eating. You don't want to overcompensate on the days before fasting either by eating more calories in an effort to make up for the upcoming calorie restriction.

And as you learned earlier, you must be in a caloric deficit to lose weight, so that's the top priority. The 5:2 diet is simply the sustainable method by which you'll create your caloric deficit. Later on, I'll share with you how you can measure the amount of calories you're eating to ensure you stay on track.

Chapter 5: How to Eat on Fasting Days

The guidelines for fasting days seems simple enough—eat 500 calories for the day if you're a female and 600 for the day if you're a male. However, there are different ways to consume your 500-600 calories, and you can experiment to find which pattern works best for you. The following are the two typical patterns that people will follow on their fasting days:

-Three small meals: Typically you'll eat a breakfast, lunch, and dinner, each consisting of about 167-200 calories.

Or:

-Two slightly larger meals: With this option, you'll skip breakfast and eat only lunch and dinner. Each meal will consist of around 250-300 calories.

Either option will work, however I prefer the second option where you only eat two meals. By eating three meals per day, you're increasing your chances of overeating during one of those meals. Each meal only consists of 200 calories or less, which is really more along the lines of a snack and not meal. If you're extra hungry, you might continue to eat beyond the calories you're allowed to eat for that meal, which would hinder your results.

By only eating two meals per day, you'll get to enjoy slightly larger meals. Plus you'll skip breakfast entirely, which will allow you to not even have to think about food until later in the day. This will also lessen the chances of you overeating.

What Should You Eat for Your Meals?

With only 500-600 calories allowed on your fasting days, you must be wise with how you use your calories. You'll want the majority of what you eat to come from high-quality foods that are satiating. It won't take long to reach 500-600 calories by eating junk food such as potato chips and ice cream. Additionally, these types of food won't do much to fill you up and keep you full.

You'll want the majority of your diet to consist of foods high in protein and fiber. Fiber and protein will help to get you feeling full for long periods of time without having to consume a lot of calories. Plus, protein has the highest thermic effect of food of the three macronutrients.

The thermic effect of food is simply the amount of energy required to eat, digest, absorb, and store food. Essentially, your body burns calories to digest the foods you eat!

Here's the approximate TEF for each macronutrient:

- Protein: 30-35%
- Carbs: 5-15%
- Fat: 3-4%

This means that if you consume 100 calories from protein, your body will burn roughly 30-35 calories to digest and process those original 100 calories. Conversely, if you consumed 100 calories from carbs, your body would only burn about 5-15 calories to digest and process the original 100 calories.

And since your calories are being restricted on your fasting days, it makes sense to consume high amounts of protein to maximize the TEF effect.

Specific Foods to Eat on Your Fasting Days

The following is a list of high-quality foods and drinks that you can consume on your fasting days to help keep you full even though your calories are being restricted:

- Vegetables
- Lean Meat
- Boiled Eggs
- Fish
- Protein Powder
- Cauliflower Rice
- Cottage Cheese
- Black coffee
- Tea

The cool thing about this dieting approach is that it'll allow you to be able to eat your favorite foods from time to time. However, on your fasting days I strongly recommend that you eat healthy foods high in fiber and protein. You'll also want to keep healthy fats at a bare minimum.

Yes, foods like almonds, olive oil, and avocados are healthy for you, but fat contains 9 calories per gram opposed to carbs and protein, which only contain 4 calories per gram. This means that calories you consume from fat will add up more than twice as fast as calories consumed from carbs and protein.

It's not mandatory for you to consume low amounts of fat and no junk food on your fasting days. However, if you want to see the best success possible with the 5:2 diet, then you'll want to stick to the guidelines I mentioned above.

What to Do If You Feel Irritable or Extremely Hungry

If you've never done any type of fasting protocol before, then you must be patient and give your body time to adjust to this new style of eating. Far too many people quit after a few days because it's too difficult. Yes, the first few times of fasting will be hard, but that's because you're body hasn't adapted to this eating pattern yet. If you've lived your whole life eating a standard breakfast, lunch, and dinner, do you think your body is expecting you to suddenly eat 500-600 calories a day twice per week? No way.

It takes time for us to adjust to new things. Imagine getting a new job or moving to a different city. It might be a little awkward at first, but as time goes on you'll get used to your new environment. Your body is no different. Of course I understand that being patient is easier said than done when you're unbelievably hungry, but don't worry, the following tips will help to make the adjustment phase easier.

Tip #1: Understand that fasting isn't for everyone.

Yes, I'm a really big fan of fasting, but I understand that it's not for everyone. Fasting is simply one approach to help you get and stay lean for life. There are other nutrition strategies out there that will work—fasting may be it for you, and it may not be. You'll never know unless you try. The best diet is the one that works for you and allows you to stay in a caloric deficit for a long period of time. Don't beat yourself up or feel guilty if in the end fasting isn't the right fit for you.

Tip #2: Do the 5:2 diet for at least two weeks

The reason why you'll want to do the 5:2 diet for at least two weeks is because that's about how long it'll take your body to get used to it. If you give up on it before then, how do you know if it was really right for you? Was it not a good fit, or did your body not have enough time to get used to it? You'll never know unless you actually give the diet a chance to work.

Tip #3: Chew gum during your fasting days

Chewing sugar free gum on your fasting days can act as a really good way to distract yourself while you're hungry. Keep a pack of gum on you at all times so you can easily chew a piece whenever you start to feel irritable or ravenously hungry.

Tip #4: Drink black coffee

Research shows that coffee can act as a good appetite suppressant (9). Drink one to two cups of coffee in the morning or throughout the day to help blunt some of the hunger you might be feeling. The key is though that it needs to be plain black coffee. Adding milk, creamer, and sugar will not only dissipate the fasting benefits, but also add up in calories very quickly. When you're limited to 500-600 calories a day, the last thing you want to do is waste them on beverages that won't keep you full.

Tip #5: Stay hydrated

Sometimes your body will play tricks on you. It'll make you think that you're hungry when in reality you're dehydrated and your body is confusing thirst for hunger. Anytime you're hungry and you think it might be false hunger, drink 1-2 glasses of water, wait 10 minutes and see how you feel. If you're still hungry after that waiting period, then you could actually be hungry. But if not, drinking water could've saved you from eating unnecessary calories due to false hunger.

Tip #6: Stay Busy

As I mentioned earlier, you'll want to plan your fasting days for when you're the busiest. If all you're doing is sitting around thinking about how hungry you are, you're going to cave. That's why it's a good idea to put your fasting days on weekdays when you have work and potentially have other activities to keep you busy. On weekends you might want to have a nice dinner with your friends and family, and fasting on those days would prevent you from being able to do so.

Chapter 6: How to Eat on Non-Fasting Days

On non-fasting days, you're supposed to eat how you normally would. This answer works fine for some people, but others want to have a bit more structure. Whatever type of person you are, don't worry; I'll be covering both options.

Whether you prefer to have more flexibility or more structure, remember that you must be in a caloric deficit. Even if you're eating 500-600 calories twice per week, that alone doesn't guarantee weight loss. You must consistently be in a caloric deficit on a weekly basis in order to get the scale moving. Sure, you might be in a caloric deficit on your fasting days, but if you're overeating on your non-fasting days, it could offset your calories enough to prevent weight loss. Make sure you follow that rule above anything else.

How to Eat if You Prefer More Flexibility

If you like the idea of having more flexibility on your fasting days, then you can pretty much eat how you please (within reason of course) and do what works best for you. As far as meal frequency is concerned, eat as many meals as you like. A common myth is that eating more frequently throughout the day will boost your metabolism.

This is how eating six meals a day became so popular. However, research shows that meal frequency doesn't matter for weight loss (10). Calorie volume is what matters for weight loss. Therefore you can eat one, three, or even six meals per day and weight loss will be the same as long as the total amount of calories you're eating is in check.

This should come as a relief to you. It's not going to be easy to consistently consume six meals a day if you have a busy schedule. So simply eat as frequently as you like. Another thing you can do is disperse your allotted calories between your meals however you like. For example, let's say you're eating 1,500 calories on your non-fasting days, and you're eating three meals a day.

Most people prefer to keep things easy and disperse their calories evenly between those three meals. In this instance that would mean eating 500 calories for your first, second, and third meal. However, let's say you like eating larger meals later in the day. You could sacrifice calories on your first and/or second meal to allow you more calories for your third and final meal that you'll be eating later in the day.

Here are a couple of examples of how you could break up your total calories. We'll use the example from above and pretend your total daily calories is 1,500:

Example #1:

Meal #1: 250 calories
Meal #2: 250 calories
Meal #3: 1,000 calories

Example #2:

Meal #1: 150 calories
Meal #2: 550 calories
Meal #3: 800 calories

Of course you can mix and match your calories between meals however you like. It's a good idea to plan ahead. For example, you might have an upcoming wedding that you'll be attending. In that case, you'll want to save as many calories as you can for the wedding. You won't want to miss out on all of the amazing foods that'll be there, and you won't want to mess up your diet and overeat.

And there might be another instance where you're at a really good bed and breakfast. Go ahead and enjoy eating a nice breakfast while you're there and simply eat less calories than usual for your remaining meals.

Also, you don't have to be super diligent about tracking your calories if you're taking the flexible approach. Initially for the first couple of weeks or so, it is a good idea to track your calories through an app like My Fitness Pal. This will help to ensure that you're eating the correct amount of calories. It'll also give you a feel for how you need to eat on your non-fasting days to lose weight.

Once you start to get the hang of things, you'll be able to eyeball your food items and get a ballpark estimate of the amount of calories they contain. Make sure you're still measuring your weight on a weekly basis to ensure that you're still losing weight. If you're not, then you'll need to become more rigid with tracking calories or switch to a more structured approach.

As for what foods you should be eating, you can really eat as you please as long as you're eating below your resting metabolic rate (bodyweight x13=total daily calories). One of the worst dieting mistakes you can make is restricting your favorite foods. This will make the 5:2 diet far less enjoyable, and it'll make you more likely to quit and binge eat.

Instead, eat your favorite foods roughly 15% of the time and eat clean and healthy foods the other 85%. This will give you the best of both worlds. You'll get to enjoy eating whatever foods you want, and it'll allow you to enjoy special events like birthdays and parties. At the same time, you're not eating enough junk food to completely ruin any progress you're making on your fasting days. Eating healthy foods the majority of the time will keep you energized and keep you satiated. Of course, eating clean can get bland at times and that's when eating tasty treats will come in handy. In a later chapter, I'll provide you with a list of some high quality recipes you can eat.

How to Eat if You Prefer More Structure

Eating how you normally do on non-fasting days might work fine and dandy for some, but what if you want more of a planned routine that you can follow? Don't worry, I've got you covered. Here's the step-by-step process you need to follow for your non-fasting days:

Step #1: Determine your weekly calorie budget

Think of your calories like money in a bank account. Each week you have a certain amount of calories to eat, just like you have a certain budget for your finances. If you don't use your calories wisely and you overeat, you won't lose any weight. This is similar to spending money not in your budget to go shopping and then not having enough money to cover basic bills.

In order to figure this out, you'll need to use the resting metabolic rate (RMR) equation from the earlier chapter:

Bodyweight x 13= RMR

Remember your RMR is the amount of calories you'll burn off in a given day. You'll then need to multiply that number by seven to find out how many calories you're burning off in a week. Let's use myself as an example:

Bodyweight=195 pounds
195 x 13= RMR of 2,535

2,535 x 7= 17,745

This means that I burn approximately 17,745 calories in a week. At face value, this number doesn't mean much. It's hard to interpret it and understand exactly what it means. It's kind of like someone saying they lost 15 kilograms. Is that a lot or a little? It's hard to tell if you're used to pounds. Don't worry though, this number will make sense in a bit.

Step #2: Subtract Your Fasting Day Calories

The next thing you'll want to do is subtract the calories you'll be eating on your fasting days. This is going to be 500 calories for women and 600 for men. Since you'll be fasting twice per week, this means that men need to subtract 1,200 from their weekly total and women need to subtract 1,000 calories. Coming back to my example:

17,745-1,200= 16,545

This means that I'll be eating a total of about 16,545 on my five non-fasting days. The amount of calories you'll be eating on your fasting days is already set up for you, but we're going to have to dig a little deeper to find out how much we need to eat on our non-fasting days.

Step #3: Convert calories from maintenance to deficit.

The way the numbers are worked out thus far would have you eating at maintenance levels, which means that you'll neither gain nor lose weight. Not gaining weight is certainly a good thing, but it's not what we want. We want to lose weight and in order to do that we need to create a caloric deficit.

As stated earlier, there are roughly 3,500 calories in one pound of fat. This means that you'll need to create a weekly deficit of 3,500 calories or 500 calories daily in order to lose one pound per week. Losing weight at a pace of one pound per week is perfect for most people.

Imagine trying to lose 2 pounds per week, you'd have to create an average deficit of 1,000 calories a day! You might be able to sustain that for a short time, but it won't last long. Picture a year from now losing 52 pounds because you were able to diligently create an average weekly deficit of 3,500 calories! It would be hard to be upset with those results even though 1 pound per week doesn't sound glamorous.

Therefore, you'll need to take your weekly non-fasting calories and subtract 3,500 from that number. This'll take you from maintaining your bodyweight to losing one pound per week:

16,545-3,500= 13,045

Step #4: Determine daily non-fasting day calories

Now that you know your weekly non-fasting day calories, it's time to determine what that translates into on a daily basis. To figure this out, you'll simply take your weekly non-fasting day calories calculated from step three and divide that number by five. Continuing on with my example:

13,045/5= 2,609

This means that I'll need to eat 600 calories on my fasting days and 2,609 calories on my non-fasting days in order to lose approximately one pound per week. In my case, if I was normally eating more than 2,609 calories on my non-fasting days, I'd be offsetting the progress I made on my fasting days. That's why it's a good idea to know the numbers you need to hit your goal instead of winging it.

Step #5: Measure your calories

Simply knowing that you need to eat a certain amount of calories (2,609 in my case) isn't enough. Unless you're tracking how many calories you're eating then how do you know for certain? As I mentioned earlier, you'll eventually get a feel for how you need to eat to reach your target calories. Until you reach that point though, you must be strict about measuring your calories. Yes it's a pain in the neck, but you'll save time in the long run since you won't have to guess if you're on the right path.

The simplest way to do this is to go to the app or android store and download an app like My Fitness Pal or similar calorie counting app. Many of these apps have label scanners so you can simply scan a label and it'll instantly put all of the calories in that food item towards your daily budget. Plus since our smart phones are with us pretty much everywhere we go, it's easy to track your calories right then and there.

If you're unable to find the amount of calories in a food item on the app you're using, you can simply Google it or take your best guess. No matter what though, counting calories isn't going to be 100% accurate. Sometimes you'll miscalculate things and food labels aren't exact right down to the last number. Therefore, don't get frustrated if you're having trouble counting calories at first. You'll get better at it as time goes on.

Your goal is to get within 5% of your daily calories. I would drive myself insane if I had to eat 2,609 calories spot on for five days of the week. It wouldn't happen and I would give up on it soon enough. Understand that you won't be perfect either and you don't need to be. You simply have to be heading in the right direction. You can make sure you're on the right track by measuring your weight once a week.

It's best to measure your weight only once per week soon after you wake up for the most accurate results. If you measure your weight everyday, you might get discouraged because your weight may have fluctuated and gone up. You didn't actually gain any weight; you just had a fluctuation in bodyweight. By measuring once a week, you'll measure for true weight loss or gain.

If you're steadily losing about one pound per week, then great keep doing what you're doing. If it's been a couple of weeks and you still haven't lost any weight, don't give up yet. The next step will help you out...

Step #6: Make Necessary Adjustments

If you're tracking your calories, but still not seeing any process, then you may need to make some adjustments. The first thing you must check for is to make sure that you're accurately measuring your calories. Thoroughly recheck your food journal in your app by making sure you correctly logged the amount of calories in the foods you ate.

If everything checks out, then you may need to readjust your resting metabolic rate. For example, if you ate 2,000 calories on your non-fasting days and your weight stayed the same, then 2,000 calories was your true intake for maintaining your weight not losing weight. You can simply adjust this number by subtracting 250 from that original number. In this example:

2,000-250= 1,750

Now your new caloric intake on non-fasting days is 1,750 calories. You'll want to measure your weight after a week and see if you've lost any weight. If you did lose weight, then great. If not, then you'll want to go ahead and decrease that number by increments of 100 calories per week until you start losing weight. Here's how it would look:

Week 1: 2,000 calories on non-fasting days
Week 2: 2,000 calories on non-fasting days
Week 3: 1,750 calories on non-fasting days
Week 4: 1,650 calories on non-fasting days
Week 5: 1,550 calories on non-fasting days etc. until you start losing weight.

The reason why you're making such small adjustments at a time is for a couple of reasons:

1. You're probably not as far off track as you might think.
2. Easing into it will make it easier for you to adjust to your new intake instead of panicking and making drastic changes that aren't necessary.

Aside from this, there's one other tactic you can try. One common error humans make is that we tend to overestimate the amount of calories we burn from exercise, and we underestimate the amount of calories that we eat. Therefore, we can account for some of this human bias by implementing the 10% rule.

All you have to do is simply add 10% more calories to everything that you eat. For example, if you're eating a banana that your food app says is 100 calories you'll take 10% of that number and add it to the original.

100 x .1=10

10+100=110 calories

You'll now log the banana as 110 calories instead of the original 100. Do this for everything you eat and drink, no matter how many calories it contains. Adding 10% may not seem like a lot—it might even seem like a hassle, but doing this can tip the scale in your favor and account for any label inaccuracies or miscalculations.

Chapter 7: What About Exercise?

Yes the 5:2 diet is a great nutritional strategy, but you can also use it to help maximize fat loss in the gym. There are a couple of different ways to take advantage of this. The first way is by being in a fasted state when you workout. All you need to do is workout in the morning or early afternoon before you've eaten anything.

This'll be easy to achieve on your fasting days since you're only consuming 500-600 calories anyway. On your non-fasting days, you'll simply want to delay eating until you've finished your workout. Of course don't sweat it if your schedule doesn't allow for you to workout fasted, working out when you can is better than not at all.

When you workout in a fed state, your body will use the glycogen in your body as fuel for energy. However when you workout fasted, your body will be glycogen depleted. This means that your body won't be able to tap into your glycogen stores for energy, it'll have to go somewhere else. Guess where that somewhere else is? Your fat stores!

So by working out in a fasted state, your body will become more efficient at using fat for energy instead of carbs. The second thing you can do to maximize fat loss from working out is delay eating after your workout. The media has done a good job of making us think we must immediately consume protein after a workout or else it was a waste. Research shows that your body won't lose muscle if you don't eat protein within 45 minutes of your workout (11).

Whenever you workout, your body's growth hormone levels will increase (12). This growth hormone will help to protect your muscle and increase fat burning. However if you eat right after you finish a workout, your growth hormone levels will be blunted and insulin levels will increase. For this reason, you'll want to delay eating anything after finishing a workout for 1-2 hours.

Eating more calories won't help you lose more weight. Yet when it comes to eating after a workout, people act like they're immune to gaining fat from these extra calories. "I hit it hard in the gym today, I deserve a large milkshake!" No, you don't.

Imagine you go to the gym and burn 300 calories. Then, immediately after your workout, you consume a 350-calorie post workout protein shake. Now you've completely wiped out all of the calories you burned from the workout, plus you ate an additional 50 calories! It's ok to eat a meal after working out if that's when you would normally eat anyway.

Don't go out of your way to eat extra calories for the sake of a post workout shake—it won't help you burn more fat! You might be weary of working out fasted if you usually workout in a fed state. Give it a try for 1-2 weeks to give your body a chance to adapt to it. Once you do, you should notice that you have more focus and intensity in the gym.

Here's a good workout plan you can follow if you're unsure of what to do in the gym:

This regimen consists of 3 full-bodyweight workouts per week. You'll complete the same workout every time you go to the gym. You can set up your workout schedule in one of the following ways:

Monday: Workout
Tuesday: Rest
Wednesday: Workout

Thursday: Rest
Friday: Workout
Saturday: Rest
Sunday: Rest

Or

Monday: Rest
Tuesday: Workout
Wednesday: Rest
Thursday: Workout
Friday: Rest
Saturday: Workout
Sunday: Rest

Full-body workouts will provide you with many benefits:

-You'll burn more calories from your workouts.
-You'll gain strength and muscle faster since you'll be
stimulating your muscles more frequently.
-You'll have better nervous system recovery because you
won't train on consecutive days.
-You'll develop perfect form on key lifts faster because you
practice them more often.

Also, if your body has never been exposed to this stimulus
(i.e. weightlifting) before, you can take advantage of what
some people call "newbie gains." And by increasing the
frequency at which you stimulate your muscle groups, you
can speed up the process.

Side Note: A set is a group of consecutive repetitions. A
repetition is one complete motion of an exercise. And the
rest period is how long of a break you'll take until you start
the next set. For example, let's say you're completing 3 sets
of 8 reps and resting 2 minutes in between sets for the
barbell squat exercise.

You'll squat down and stand back up, completing the motion
of the exercise and one rep. You'll repeat that motion 7 more

times for a total of 8 repetitions. That will complete the set and you will begin your rest period. Once your 2-minute rest period is up, you'll start the next set and perform another 8 repetitions.

That will complete set number 2, and you'll rest another 2 minutes. Once that time period is up, you'll complete the final set of 8 repetitions, and then you'll move onto the next exercise.

Here's the workout:

- Incline Barbell Bench Press: 3 sets 8 reps 2 min rest between (btw) sets
- Barbell Back Squats: 3 sets of 8 reps 2 min rest btw sets
- Lat Pulldowns: 3 sets of 10 reps 90 sec rest btw sets
- Seated DB Military Press: 3 sets of 8 reps 2 min rest btw sets
- Standing DB Curls: 3 sets of 12 reps 60 sec rest btw sets
- Tricep Rope Pushdowns: 3 sets of 12 reps 60 sec rest btw sets

That's all there is to it! Don't let the simplicity of it fool you—it will work.

What About Cardio?

If you're looking to burn fat, cardio can definitely be a handy tool to help you out. It's a great form of exercise you can do regardless if you're into weight training or not. Cardio will do one of two things for you:

#1: Speed up the rate at which you lose fat.
Or

#2: Give you some extra leeway in your diet.

Cardio is by no means necessary for you to reach your fat loss goals, but it will help. What type of cardio should you do—slow and steady or running? Science shows that the best type of cardio you can do is something called high intensity interval training (HIIT) (13).

This kind of cardio combines high intensity cardio with low intensity cardio. HIIT by itself is very effective, but it can be maximized when you immediately follow it with slow steady state cardio. The intensity of the HIIT will release free fatty acids into your bloodstream, and the slow steady state cardio will burn them off. Here's how to perform this hybrid cardio workout:

Part 1: HIIT

Alternate between a high intensity and a low intensity for 10-15 minutes on your choice of cardio machine. Here's an example on a treadmill:
-Run at 7.5 mph for 1 minute
-Walk at 3.5 mph for 1 minute
-Repeat for 10-15 minutes

Part 2: Slow steady state cardio (done immediately after HIIT)

Example on a treadmill: Walk at a constant pace of 3.5-4 mph for 10-15 minutes

Note: If you need to adjust the intensity of the HIIT then do so. You can alter the run-walk ratios (i.e. run for 30 seconds and walk for 1.5 minutes), or you can decrease the intensity of each run (i.e. run at 6 mph instead of 7.5). And if what I prescribed is too easy, then ramp up the intensity accordingly.

Yes, the 5:2 diet alone will be enough to help you start losing weight and exercise isn't mandatory for it to work. However, exercise will provide you with many additional health benefits and it'll help you lose more weight (14).

Chapter 8: 28 Low-Calorie Recipes

This chapter contains 28 recipes that are all below 200 calories per serving. These recipes are great ideas for what to eat on your fasting days because your calories will be heavily restricted on those days. I've included a wide variety of dishes including soups and even some desserts.

Of course like I mentioned earlier, you'll want to be cautious eating desserts on your fasting days and it's probably best to save those recipes for your non-fasting days. Enjoy!

Five Ingredient Soup

Ingredients:

- 1 can of fat-free chicken broth
- 1 can of corn
- 1 can of black beans
- 1 can of fat-free refried beans
- 1 can of diced tomatoes

*All can sizes are 14.4 ounces

Directions:

Combine ingredients into medium saucepan.
Whisk to integrate refried beans.
Simmer then serve.
Garnish as desired.

Number of servings: 10

Macros (per serving):

Calories: 128.0
Protein: 7.3 g
Carbs: 24.9 g
Fat: 0.6 g

French Onion Soup

Ingredients:

- ¼ cup of water
- 1 medium onion
- 4 cups of beef broth
- ½ cup shredded part-skim mozzarella cheese

Directions:

1. Bring water to boil in medium saucepan.
2. Slice onions into thin strips and add to water.
3. Continue cooking until onions clarify.
4. When onions are translucent, add in the beef broth.
5. Bring to boil and simmer for 15-20 minutes.
6. Once done, add in the mozzarella cheese and enjoy!

Number of servings: 2

Macros (per serving):

Calories: 165.9
Protein: 14.6 g
Carbs: 14.7 g
Fat: 6.1 g

Cabbage Vegetable Soup

Ingredients:

- 1, 28 oz can of crushed tomatoes
- 1 medium diced onion
- 3 stalks of diced celery
- 1 shredded head of cabbage
- 1, 14.5 oz can of green beans
- 1, 12 oz can of sweet yellow corn
- 1, 15 oz can of pinto beans

Directions:

1. Place tomatoes, onion, celery, carrots, and cabbage in a pot
2. Simmer over medium heat until tender for about 20 minutes.
3. Add in the canned vegetables.
4. Heat, serve, and enjoy!

Number of servings: 6

Macros (per serving):

Calories: 165.2
Protein: 8.3 g
Carbs: 36.6 g
Fat: 1.8 g

Butternut Squash and Apple Soup

Ingredients:

- 2 tbsp. unsalted butter
- 1 medium chopped yellow onion
- 1 butternut squash, about 3 lbs., peeled, seeded & cut into 1" cubes
- 6 cups low-sodium chicken broth
- 4 medium peeled, cored, and chopped Granny Smith apples
- 1/4 tsp. freshly ground nutmeg
- 4 pinches of Spanish saffron threads, about 1 tsp. or 1 tsp. sweet curry
- 2 cups fat-free half & half
- Salt and pepper to taste

Directions:

1. In a large soup pot, over medium heat, melt butter and sauté' onion until tender, for 4 to 6 minutes.
2. Add the squash and broth, bring to a boil and reduce heat to medium-low.
   Simmer, stirring occasionally, until the squash is tender when pierced with a fork.
3. Add chopped apples, saffron or curry (if desired) and nutmeg.
4. Simmer until the apples are tender, stirring occasionally. Using a food processor or blender, puree the soup in batches until smooth.
5. Return the soup to the pot and stir in half and half. Season, to taste with salt and pepper.

Number of servings: 12

Macros (per serving):

Calories: 135.3
Protein: 3.9 g

Carbs: 25.8 g
Fat: 3.1 g

Beef Vegetable Soup

Ingredients:

- 2 cups of canned tomatoes
- 1 cups of cabbage
- 3-4 sliced carrots
- 2 cups of green beans
- ½ cup of celery
- 1 lb. of stew beef

Directions:

1. Cook meat until tender with 1-2 tbsp. of oil.
2. Combine all vegetables with cooked meat.
3. Season with 1 tsp. of salt and simmer for 1 hour.
4. Add in broth or tomato juice for additional liquid as needed.

Number of servings: 6

Macros (per serving):

Calories: 192.3
Protein: 22.1 g
Carbs: 18.5 g
Fat: 3.6 g

Tomato Soup

Ingredients:

- 2 tbsp. olive oil
- 1 yellow or white onion, chopped (about 1 cup)
- 3 cloves garlic, minced
- 2 pounds of deseeded and chopped tomatoes
- 1/4 tsp. red pepper flakes
- 1 tbsp. brown sugar
- 1/2 teaspoon dried thyme
- 4 small slices whole-wheat bread, crust removed
- 1 1/2 cups low-sodium chicken or vegctable stock
- 1 tbsp. balsamic vinegar
- Pepper to taste

Directions:

1. Heat oil in large saucepan.
2. Add in the onions and garlic and sauté for 5 minutes.
3. Stir in the tomatoes; add in the pepper, sugar, thyme and bread and cook for 3 minutes.
4. Puree using a food processor.
5. Slowly add the stock and simmer for 10 minutes. Add in the vinegar and cook for another 2 minutes.

Number of servings: 8

Macros (per serving):

Calories: 98.9
Protein: 2.5 g
Carbs: 14.3 g
Fat: 4.1 g

Chicken Noodle Soup

Ingredients:

- 1 package fettuccine noodles
- 1 cup chopped onion
- 1 cup chopped cabbage
- 1 cup spinach
- 1 cup chopped carrots
- 1 clove garlic
- 1 tsp. ginger
- 1 tsp. red pepper flakes
- 8 oz. chicken
- 4 cups broth
- 1 tbsp. soy sauce

Directions:

1. Rinse fettuccini noodles under warm water for 30 seconds, drain, and let air dry while preparing other ingredients.
2. Boil the 4 cups of broth.
3. Add all of the ingredients to the broth (noodles included) and cook for 6-7 minutes until vegetables become tender.

Number of servings: 4

Macros (per serving):

Calories: 174.5
Protein: 18.8 g
Carbs: 11.8 g
Fat: 6.1 g

Tuna Salad

Ingredients:

- 1 can albacore tuna
- 2/3 cup non-fat cottage cheese
- 4 tbsp. plain low-fat yogurt
- 1/4 small red onion, finely chopped
- 1 stalk celery, finely chopped
- 1 tsp. Dijon mustard
- Squirt of lemon juice
- A pinch of dill

Directions:

1. Mix all of the ingredients in a bowl and enjoy!

Number of servings: 2

Macros (per serving):

Calories: 190.3
Protein: 32.5 g
Carbs: 11.7 g
Fat: 2.2 g

Parmesan Shrimp

Ingredients:

- 14 medium shrimp, peeled and deveined
- 1 tbsp. olive oil
- 1/2 clove garlic, minced
- 2 dashes of salt
- 1/4 tsp. Creole seasoning
- 2 dashes of ground pepper
- 1/8 cup Panko breadcrumbs
- 1 tbsp. shredded parmesan cheese

Directions:

1. Place shrimp, garlic, olive oil, salt, pepper and Creole seasoning into Ziploc bag.
2. Flip bag in multiple directions until shrimp is well coated.
3. Place in fridge for 1.5 hours.
4. Preheat oven to 475 degrees F.
5. Add bread crumbs and Parmesan to bag and turn until coated.
6. Spray a baking pan with butter and arrange shrimp on pan to where they don't touch.
7. Broil for roughly 10 minutes or until thoroughly cooked.
8. Add in the squeezed lemon and enjoy!

Number of servings: 2

Macros (per serving):

Calories: 137.6
Protein: 10.2 g
Carbs: 4.7 g
Fat: 8.6 g

Crustless Quiche

Ingredients:

- 1 cup non-fat cottage cheese
- 2 cups liquid egg whites
- 1/2 cup cooled broccoli
- 1/2 cup ham
- 1/2 cup low-fat Colby cheese
- Salt and pepper to taste

Directions:

1. Preheat oven to 375 degrees F.
2. Mix all of the ingredients into a large bowl.
3. Spray a pie dish with cooking spray.
4. Put mixture into pie dish.
5. Put dish into oven, bake for 45 minutes and enjoy!

Number of servings: 6

Macros (per serving):

Calories: 106.8
Protein: 18.7 g
Carbs: 4.5 g
Fat: 1.4 g

Salmon Cakes

Ingredients:

- 1 can wild Alaskan Pink Salmon
- 1 cup raw onion
- 1 tsp. black pepper
- 1 tsp. garlic powder
- 1 large egg
- salt to taste

Directions:

1. Mix all of the ingredients together.
2. For mixture into 4 separate patties.
3. Fry patties similar to the way you would a burger until thoroughly cooked.

Number of servings: 4

Macros (per serving):

Calories: 195.0
Protein: 23.2 g
Carbs: 4.5 g
Fat: 10.1 g

Regular Chicken Salad

Ingredients:

- 1 1/2 cups cooked and chopped chicken
- 1 1/2 cups chopped celery
- 3 tbsp. light mayonnaise
- 1 tsp. mustard
- Salt and pepper to taste

Directions:

1. Put all of the ingredients together in a bowl and thoroughly mix together.

Number of servings: 1

Macros (per serving):

Calories: 173.8
Protein: 24.2 g
Carbs: 3.5 g
Fat: 6.3 g

Lettuce Wraps

Ingredients:

- 3.5 oz. lean ground beef
- 1 tbsp. finely minced onion
- 1 clove crushed minced garlic
- Dash garlic powder
- Dash dried oregano
- Chopped cilantro to taste
- Cayenne pepper to taste
- Salt and pepper to taste
- Lettuce leaves

Directions:

1. Brown ground beef until thoroughly cooked.
2. Add onion, garlic, spices, and a little water and simmer for 7-10 minutes.
3. Add salt to taste.
4. Add mixture onto lettuce, wrap it up, and enjoy!

Number of servings: 1

Macros (per serving):

Calories: 143.5
Protein: 21.7 g
Carbs: 4.2 g
Fat: 1.4 g

Country Style Crockpot Pork Ribs

Ingredients:

- 1/4 tsp. ground allspice
- 1/4 tsp. ground cinnamon
- 2 pounds country-style pork ribs
- 1/4 cup diced onion
- 1/2 tsp. garlic powder
- 1 tbsp. sugar-free maple-flavored syrup
- 1 dash black pepper
- 1/4 tsp. ground ginger
- 1 tbsp. low-sodium soy sauce

Directions:

1. Mix all of the ingredients into a bowl minus the ribs.
2. Pour mixture over ribs.
3. Put ribs in crockpot and cook for 8-9 hours on low.
4. Cover with foil and bake for 60-90 minutes if baking in oven.

Number of servings: 4

Macros (per serving):

Calories: 188.4
Protein: 22.3 g
Carbs: 2.3 g
Fat: 9.4 g

Tuna Burgers

Ingredients:

- 2 cups tuna
- 1/3 cup tomato sauce
- 1/4 cup finely chopped dill pickle onions
- 2 egg whites
- 1/4 cup wholegrain flour
- 1/4 tsp. black pepper
- 1/2 tsp. garlic powder
- 1/2 tsp. onion powder

Directions:

1. Put all of the ingredients in a bowl and thoroughly mix together.
2. Form mixture into 4 separate patties.
3. Spray skillet with cooking spray and cook on medium-high heat until thoroughly cooked on each side.
4. Serve and enjoy!

Number of servings: 4

Macros (per serving):

Calories: 140.5
Protein: 23.7 g
Carbs: 8.5 g
Fat: 1.3 g

Scampi Shrimp

Ingredients:

- 1 tbsp. canola oil
- 3/4 lb. uncooked peeled and deveined shrimp
- 1 med diced green onion
- 1/4 tsp. garlic powder
- 1/2 tsp. basil
- 3/4 tsp. parsley
- 1 tbsp. lemon juice
- 3 tbsp. parmesan cheese

Directions:

1. Heat oil over medium heat in 10" skillet.
2. Add shrimp and remaining ingredients to skillet.
3. Cook for 5-7 minutes.
4. Remove skillet from heat and sprinkle with Parmesan cheese.
5. Serve and enjoy!

Number of servings: 4

Macros (per serving):

Calories: 143.5
Protein: 19.0 g
Carbs: 2.1 g
Fat: 6.1 g

No-Carb Cajun Tilapia

Ingredients:

- 4 oz. tilapia filet
- 1 tsp. extra virgin olive oil
- 1/2 tbsp. unsalted butter
- Favorite Cajun spice of your choosing to taste

Directions:

1. Melt butter and olive oil in a skillet.
2. Cover fish with Cajun spice.
3. Cook fish fillet in butter and oil for 3-5 minutes per side until thoroughly cooked.
4. Serve and enjoy!

Number of servings: 1

Macros (per serving):

Calories: 143.9
Protein: 21.0 g
Carbs: 0.0 g
Fat: 6.3 g

Cauliflower Faux Mashed Potatoes

Ingredients:

- 1 head raw cauliflower (5-6 in. in diameter)
- 1/4 cup sour cream
- 2 tbsp. salted butter

Directions:

1. Steam cauliflower until soft.
2. Put cooked cauliflower in a pot and heat to get rid of the excess moisture.
3. Puree cauliflower in food processor.
4. Add butter and sour cream and enjoy!

Number of servings: 4

Macros (per serving):

Calories: 117.6
Protein: 3.4 g
Carbs: 8.1 g
Fat: 9.1 g

Dinner Rolls

Ingredients:

- 1/4 cup honey
- 1 cup warm water
- 1 envelope yeast
- 1/3 cup non-fat dry milk
- 1/3 cup unsalted melted butter
- 2 eggs
- 1 tsp. salt
- 4 1/2 cups flour

Directions:

1. Dissolve honey and yeast in warm water and let it stand until foamy.
2. Add in the milk powder, butter, eggs and salt then stir.
3. Gradually add in the flour and knead for 8 minutes.
4. Let the dough rise until doubled in height, press them down again and let them rise for 30 minutes before putting them in the oven.
5. Form into 30 round rolls and place them on the baking sheet.
6. Bake in the oven at 375 degrees F for 15 minutes.
7. Let cool for 10 minutes, serve and enjoy!

Number of servings: 30

Macros (per serving):

Calories: 80.5
Protein: 2.3 g
Carbs: 14.8 g
Fat: 1.2 g

Chicken Enchiladas

Ingredients:

- 2 skinless chicken breasts
- 1 can cream chicken soup
- 1 can cream mushroom soup
- 1/4 cup diced green chilies
- 1 cup salsa verde
- 1/4 cup chopped tomatoes
- 8 whole-wheat tortillas
- 2 cups Colby jack cheese

Directions:

1. Preheat oven to 350 degrees F.
2. Boil the chicken breast and shred when cooled.
3. Mix cream chicken and cream mushroom soups, cheese, chilies, salsa verde and tomatoes together in large bowl.
4. Remove half of the mixture from the bowl and set aside for later use.
5. Add shredded chicken remaining mixture in bowl.
6. Lay a tortilla flat and fill with about 3 tsp. of the chicken, then repeat this process for the remaining tortillas.
7. Pour the rest of the mixture you set aside earlier over the top of the enchiladas and bake for 45 minutes.
8. Cool for 15 minutes and enjoy!

Number of servings: 8
Macros (per serving):

Calories: 155.4
Protein: 13.9 g
Carbs: 4.2 g
Fat: 7.3 g

Protein Shake

Ingredients:

- 1 scoop (roughly 33 grams) vanilla cream whey protein powder
- 8 oz. unsweetened almond breeze vanilla almond milk
- 6 ice cubes
- 1 tsp. of vanilla extract

Directions:

1. Put all of the ingredients together in a blender and blend until smooth.

Number of servings: 1

Macros (per serving):

Calories: 170.0
Protein: 24.0 g
Carbs: 8.0 g
Fat: 4.5 g

Veggie Bacon Cheese Omlet

Ingredients:

- 1/4 cup liquid egg whites
- 1/4 cup raw onions
- 1/4 cup chopped green peppers
- 1/4 cup chopped tomatoes
- 1/4 cup reduced fat feta cheese
- 1/4 serving pre-cooked bacon

Directions:

1. Spray skillet with cooking spray and place on medium heat.
2. Add in peppers and onions and sauté for a bit until crisp.
3. Tear apart the bacon and add to skillet.
4. Add in the egg mixture and mix together with other ingredients.
5. Put the tomatoes and feta cheese on top and continue stirring until done.

Number of servings: 1

Macros (per serving):

Calories: 170.3
Protein: 20.3 g
Carbs: 9.6 g
Fat: 4.9 g

Teriyaki Meatballs

Ingredients:

- 1 lb. lean ground beef
- 1/2 cup chopped green onions
- 1/3 cup teriyaki sauce
- 3 tsp. chopped ginger root

Directions:

1. Preheat oven to 350 degrees F.
2. Mix all of the ingredients together in a separate bowl.
3. Form 8- 2 oz. balls with the mixture.
4. Place the balls into a dish and bake for 25-30 minutes.

Number of servings: 8

Macros (per serving):

Calories: 101.1
Protein: 13.1 g
Carbs: 3.8 g
Fat: 3.5 g

Ham and Green Bean Dinner

Ingredients:

- 2 lbs. quarter ham roast
- 6 medium sized potatoes
- 12 oz. can green beans
- 1 cup ginger ale

Directions:

1. Preheat oven to 450 degrees F.
2. Put ham roast on a baking pan and add one cup of ginger ale.
3. Place potatoes on separate pan and bake them at the same time as the ham roast.
4. Bake for about 35 minutes or until thoroughly cooked.
5. Boil the green beans while the ham roast and potatoes are baking on medium heat.
6. Serve and enjoy!

Number of servings: 6

Macros (per serving):

Calories: 190.7
Protein: 8.4 g
Carbs: 36.4 g
Fat: 1.5 g

Pumpkin Spice Frappuccino

Ingredients:

- 3/4 tsp. pumpkin spice
- 1-2 tsp. instant coffee
- 3 tbsp. canned pumpkin
- 1 tsp. stevia
- 2 tsp. sugar twin
- 3 tbsp. French vanilla coffee creamer
- 1 cup unsweetened coconut milk
- 6 ice cubes

Directions:

1. Put all of the ingredients in a blender and blend until mixture is smooth.

Number of servings: 2

Macros (per serving):

Calories: 66.3
Protein: 0.6 g
Carbs: 3.3 g
Fat: 4.7 g

Chocolate Cheesecake

Ingredients:

For Sauce:
- 2 tbsp. butter
- 4 tbsp. cocoa
- 3 tbsp. Splenda

For Cake:
- 16 oz. cream cheese
- 1 pkg. of sugar free instant chocolate pudding mix
- 1/2 cup of heavy cream
- 1/2 cup of Splenda
- 1 tsp. vanilla extract
- 2 eggs

Directions:

For Sauce:

1. Melt together butter, cocoa and Splenda (3 tbsp. worth) on stovetop or in microwave.

For Cake:

1. Preheat oven to 350 degrees F.
2. Mix together cream cheese, Splenda, vanilla and eggs.
3. Mix heavy cream and pudding together in separate bowl from other mixture.
4. Combine both mixtures toughly in blender.
5. Spray a pie plate with cooking spray.
6. Put cheesecake mixture in pan and place in oven for around 40 minutes.
7. Remove and drizzle sauce on top. Refrigerate, serve cold and enjoy!

Number of servings: 12

Macros (per serving):

Calories: 207.7
Protein: 4.8 g
Carbs: 5.4 g
Fat: 20.0 g

Snicker doodle Cookies

Ingredients:

- 1/2 cup butter
- 1 1/2 cup almond flour
- 1 cup Splenda
- 1 egg
- 1/2 tsp. vanilla
- 1/4 tsp. baking soda
- 1/4 tsp. cream of tartar
- 2 tbs. Splenda
- 1 tsp. cinnamon

Directions:

1. Mix together all of the ingredients minus the cinnamon and Splenda.
2. Cover the bowl and refrigerate for 1 hour.
3. In a separate bowl, mix together the cinnamon and Splenda.
4. Roll dough in small balls throughout Splenda and cinnamon mixture.
5. Place dough balls on mixture and bake in oven at 350 degrees F for 15 minutes.
6. Remove and cool for 10 minutes and enjoy!

Number of servings: 20

Macros (per serving):

Calories: 99.1
Protein: 2.5 g
Carbs: 4.4 g
Fat: 9.4 g

Chocolate Chip Cookies

Ingredients:

- 2 1/2 cups white flour
- 3/4 cup granulated sugar
- 3 cups old fashioned Quaker oats
- 2 cups chopped walnuts
- 2 cups chocolate chips
- 2 sticks margarine butter
- 1 tsp. salt
- 1 tsp. baking soda
- 1 cup whey protein powder
- 1 tsp. vanilla flavoring
- 3 eggs

Directions:

1. Preheat oven to 350 degrees F
2. Cream the sugars and margarine butter.
3. Add in vanilla and eggs and beat until smooth.
4. Add in protein powder then salt, baking powder, and flour and mix until smooth.
5. Add in the chocolate chips, oatmeal and walnuts and stir until smooth.
6. Use a ¼ measuring cup to portion the dough and make each cookie roughly 3" in diameter and ½" high.
7. Bake for around 10 minutes until golden brown.
8. Let them sit and cool and enjoy!

Number of servings: 48

Macros (per serving):

Calories: 168.6
Protein: 6.5 g
Carbs: 18.8 g

Fat: 8.7 g

Chapter 9: 22 High-Protein Recipes

The majority of the following recipes contain over 20 grams of protein per serving, and all of the recipes contain over 10 grams of protein. You can certainly eat some of these recipes on your fasting days. However, some of them are quite high in calories, and I would recommend saving those recipes for your non-fasting days. Enjoy!

Macaroni and Cheese Tuna Casserole

Ingredients:

- 1 box Kraft Mac N Cheese
- 1/4 cup skim milk
- 3 tsp. margarine
- 1 can tuna

Directions:

1. Boil the mac n cheese for about 8 minutes according to the box's instructions.
2. Drain the pasta.
3. Add in 1/4 cup of skim milk and stir.
4. Add in 3 tsp. of margarine and stir.
5. Add in the packet of cheese that comes with the macaroni and mix it in well.
6. Flake the tuna in the can with a fork and then add it to the macaroni and stir well.

Number of servings: 4

Macros (per serving):

Calories: 333.2
Protein: 27.6 g
Carbs: 39.8 g
Fat: 5.6 g

Venison Pot Roast

Ingredients:

- 2 1/2 lbs. venison
- 1/2 tsp. black pepper
- 1/4 tsp. salt
- 2 sliced large onions
- 1 3/4 cup water
- 1 packet onion soup mix
- 1 1/2 tbsp. balsamic vinegar
- 1 tsp. dried thyme
- 8 medium red potatoes
- 2 cups baby carrots

Directions:

1. Preheat oven to 350 degrees F.
2. Coat a pot with cooking spray and heat over medium heat.
3. Put the roast in the pan and sprinkle with salt and pepper and then place the onions around the roast.
4. Cook the roast and onions for roughly 8 minutes until they brown.
5. Add water into the pot and then stir in the soup mix, vinegar, and thyme and bring to a boil.
6. Move the roast and onions to a 9x13 pan and bake in the oven for 1 hour.
7. Put the potatoes and carrots around the roast, then cover and bake for another 2 hours until the vegetables are tender.
8. Finally, put the roast on a cutting board and slice it against the grain, then serve and enjoy!

Number of servings: 10

Macros (per serving):

Calories: 292.9
Protein: 29.4 g
Carbs: 33.0 g
Fat: 2.3 g

Turkey Tenderloin Stir Fry

Ingredients:

- 8 oz. diced turkey cutlets
- 2 cups chopped Swiss chard
- 3 cloves garlic
- 1 medium onion
- 1 cup chopped green bell peppers
- 1 cup chopped mushrooms
- 1/2 cup chopped water chestnuts
- 1 cup chopped broccoli
- 3 tbsp. soy sauce
- 1/2 cup chicken broth
- 6 tsp. granulated sugar
- 2 tbsp. cornstarch
- 1 tbsp. peanut oil
- 3 tsp. ginger root

Directions:

1. Heat oil in pan and cook peppers and onions until lightly cooked.
2. Throw in the garlic and cook for a few additional minutes.
3. Cook the turkey tenderloins until golden brown.
4. Throw in the vegetables and sauté until lightly cooked.
5. Mix together the soy sauce, cornstarch, and chicken broth. Add this mixture to the stir-fry and cook until it slightly thickens.

Number of servings: 2

Macros (per serving):

Calories: 396.1
Protein: 34.5 g
Carbs: 51.1 g

Fat: 8.1 g

Calamari Salad

Ingredients:

For Salad:
- 3 cups tossed salad
- 1 large hardboiled egg, sliced in half
- 1/2 avocado
- 4 tbsp. shredded cheddar cheese
- 1 cubic inch crumbled feta cheese
- 8 pieces sun dried tomato

For Salad Garnish and Dressing:
- 2 lemon wedges
- 2 tsp. of olive oil
- Salt and pepper to taste

For Squid:
- 200 grams raw squid
- Salt and black pepper to taste
- 2 tsp. olive oil

Directions:

1. Slice the squid into rings, place in a bowl and drizzle with 2 tsp. of olive oil.
2. Add in salt and pepper, toss around to coat and let sit for 5 minutes.
3. Divide salad ingredients on two plates, using any other veggies you like.
4. Heat a skillet on medium heat and dump squid mixture onto skillet, sautéing for 7-10 minutes.
5. Divide squid on two plates and drizzle one tsp. of olive on each plate. Add salt and pepper and a lemon wedge to each and enjoy!

Number of servings: 2

Macros (per serving):

Calories: 418.5
Protein: 28.1 g
Carbs: 19.6 g
Fat: 26.6 g

Beef Spaghetti

Ingredients:

- 1 lb. lean ground beef
- 1/2 chopped onion
- 1/2 chopped green pepper
- 10 oz. drained canned mushrooms
- 28 oz. can diced tomatoes
- 8 oz. spaghetti, broken into 1-inch pieces
- 1 cup water
- 1 1/2 tsp. Italian seasoning
- Salt and pepper to taste

Directions:

1. In a large saucepan, brown the beef and onions over medium heat until the meat is no longer pink.
2. Throw in the green pepper and mushrooms and cook for a few more minutes.
3. Then add in the diced tomatoes, spaghetti and water and stir the mixture.
4. Add in the spices.
5. Cook and cover for 15 minutes, stirring occasionally or finish when spaghetti is tender.

Number of servings: 6

Macros (per serving):

Calories: 388.5
Protein: 21.1 g
Carbs: 38.7 g
Fat: 16.5 g

Crockpot Turkey Dinner

Ingredients:

- 3/4 lb. turkey breast
- 1 can Campbell's cream of chicken soup
- 1/2 pkg. dry French onion soup mix
- 2 1/4 cup water
- 1 cup dry pearled barley
- 3 cups frozen green beans

Directions:

1. Put the turkey, soup mixes and 3/4 cup of water into the crockpot and cook on low for 6 hours.
2. After 6 hours have passed, add in the barley, remaining water and green beans, and continue cooking in the crockpot for an additional hour.
3. Serve and enjoy!

Number of servings: 6

Macros (per serving):

Calories: 328.0
Protein: 37.1 g
Carbs: 38.2 g
Fat: 2.5 g

Sausage and Black Beans

Ingredients:

- 1 tbsp. flour
- 2- 15 oz. cans black beans
- 2- 10 oz. packages frozen kernel corn
- 16 oz. jar chunky salsa
- 1 lb. smoked sliced sausage
- 1 cup Colby jack cheese

Directions:

1. Preheat oven to 450 degrees F.
2. In a large bowl, mix together the flour, beans, corn, salsa and sliced sausage.
3. Put the mixed ingredients in a large, extra heavy-duty foil bag in a 1-inch deep pan, arranged in an even layer.
4. Double fold the bag and seal it
5. Bake in the oven for 50-60 minutes.
6. Once done, hold the bag with mitts and cut it open with a knife.
7. Cautiously, fold back the top of the bag so the steam can escape.
8. Sprinkle with cheese, serve, and enjoy!

Number of servings: 5

Macros (per serving):

Calories: 546.4
Protein: 33.3 g
Carbs: 69.8 g
Fat: 14.9 g

Beef Hamburger

Ingredients:

- 6 oz. lean ground beef
- 1 hamburger bun
- 1 tbsp. light mayonnaise
- 1 tbsp. ketchup
- 1 tbsp. yellow mustard
- Toppings of your choosing

Directions:

1. Cook the ground beef on a skillet over medium heat until thoroughly cooked and there's no pink.
2. Toast the bun in a toaster.
3. Put 1 tbsp. of mayo on the bottom half of the bun.
4. Put the patty on the bottom half of the bun.
5. Add in the ketchup and mustard.
6. Put any additional toppings on the burger that you like.
7. Place the top bun on and enjoy!

Number of servings: 1

Macros (per serving):

Calories: 458.4
Protein: 38.9 g
Carbs: 26.9 g
Fat: 22.0 g

Salmon and Rice Dinner

Ingredients:

- 4 oz. wild salmon
- 1/2 cup whole grain brown rice
- 1 cup chopped broccoli
- 2 tsp. Parmesan grated cheese
- Sea salt to taste
- Garlic powder to taste
- Onion powder to taste
- Parsley to taste

Directions:

1. Preheat oven to broil.
2. Place salmon on non-stick pan with the scales facing down.
3. Season salmon with the sea salt, parsley, onion powder and garlic powder.
4. Bake the salmon for about 15 minutes.
5. While the salmon is baking, make the rice according to pkg. directions.
6. Then steam the broccoli until thoroughly heated.
7. When done, put the rice in a bowl and grate with Parmesan cheese.
8. Put rice on top of broccoli, remove the salmon and place on rice and enjoy!

Number of servings: 1

Macros (per serving):

Calories: 340.0
Protein: 29.0 g
Carbs: 32.0 g
Fat: 8.0 g

Italian Sausage and Rice

Ingredients:

- 1- 6 oz. pkg. chicken rice
- 1 lb. bulk Italian sausage
- 1 cup chopped onion
- 1 clove minced garlic
- 1 cup water
- 1- 16 oz. can peeled whole tomatoes
- 1 tsp. basil leaves
- 2 cups chopped broccoli
- 1 cup grated mozzarella cheese
- 2 tbsp. chopped parsley

Directions:

1. Brown the sausage, onion and garlic in a large skillet.
2. Add in the water, tomatoes and basil, and bring to a boil.
3. Add in the rice, reduce the heat and simmer for 15 minutes.
4. Add the broccoli and cook for another 7-10 minutes until liquid is absorbed.
5. Remove the skillet from heat, and then sprinkle with mozzarella cheese and parsley.
6. Cover and let it sit for 5 minutes, and then serve and enjoy!

Number of servings: 48

Macros (per serving):

Calories: 599.8
Protein: 29.6 g
Carbs: 38.9 g
Fat: 36.3 g

Tortellini & Bacon Dinner

Ingredients:

- 2 cups frozen tortellini
- 4 slices diced bacon
- 3 tbsp. chopped parsley
- 1 small yellow onion
- 1/2 cup Parmesan cheese
- Salt and pepper to taste

Directions:

1. Cook the frozen tortellini according to package directions and set to the side.
2. Cook the bacon until the pieces are golden brown.
3. Place the bacon bits on a paper towel to help drain the excess fat.
4. Cook the chopped onions on the same skillet used to cook the bacon until caramelized.
5. Put the bacon bits, tortellini and parsley back in and cook for another 3 minutes.
6. Next add in the Parmesan cheese and cook until it melts.
7. Serve and enjoy!

Number of servings: 4

Macros (per serving):

Calories: 230.3
Protein: 11.4 g
Carbs: 27.2 g
Fat: 8.4 g

Tilapia Parmesan

Ingredients:

- 2- 6 oz. tilapia fillets
- 2 tbsp. mayonnaise
- 2 tbsp. plain yogurt
- 1/4 cup parmesan cheese
- 3 sprigs fresh dill
- 1 tsp. garlic powder
- Black pepper to taste

Directions:

1. Put mayonnaise, yogurt and parmesan cheese in a small bowl and mix with a spoon.
2. Cover a cookie sheet with aluminum and spray with cooking spray.
3. Put oven to broil on high.
4. Put tilapia fillets roughly 2 inches apart on cookie sheet.
5. Divide cheese mixture evenly on each fillet.
6. Rub dill with fingers to separate roughly 1.5 sprigs worth of leaves over each fillet.
7. Sprinkle each fillet with half of garlic powder and season with salt and pepper.
8. Place cookie sheet into broiler.
9. Cook for 7-10 minutes, let cool and enjoy!

Number of servings: 2

Macros (per serving):

Calories: 275.2
Protein: 48.5 g
Carbs: 1.4 g
Fat: 8.5 g

Lime Chicken

Ingredients:

- 4 skinless and boneless chicken breasts
- 3 garlic cloves
- 1 cup salsa
- 1 1/2 worth lime juice
- 1/4 cup reduced fat ranch dressing
- 1 cup reduced fat cheddar cheese

Directions:

1. Spray skillet with cooking heat and place stove on medium heat.
2. Chop chicken breasts in half.
3. Sauté chicken for 3 minutes per side.
4. Add in garlic.
5. In a separate bowl, mix salsa, lime juice and ranch dressing.
6. Spread mixture onto the chicken.
7. Cook for another 5 minutes.
8. Add in the cheese and cook for another 5 minutes until chicken is no longer pink.

Number of servings: 8

Macros (per serving):

Calories: 208.9
Protein: 31.4 g
Carbs: 6.7 g
Fata: 6.2 g

Chicken Burgers

Ingredients:

- 1 lb. ground chicken
- 6 oz. crumbled feta
- 1 tbsp. ground oregano
- 1/4 tsp. salt
- 1/4 tsp. garlic powder

Directions:

1. Preheat broiler or grill.
2. Mix all of the ingredients together and form into 4 separate patties.
3. Grill or broil patties until internal temperature of burgers reaches 165 degrees F (approximately 8 minutes per side).
4. Serve and enjoy!

Number of servings: 4

Macros (per serving):

Calories: 285.6
Protein: 26.8 g
Carbs: 3.3 g
Fat: 19.8 g

Chicken Alfredo Bake

Ingredients:

- 3 boneless skinless chicken breasts
- 1 tbsp. cooking oil
- Montreal seasoning
- 1 cup cubed yellow squash
- 1 medium diced sweet onion
- 1 cup cauliflower
- salt and pepper to taste
- 1 jar Alfredo sauce
- 1/4 cup grated parmesan cheese
- 1/8 cup bread crumbs

Directions:

1. Preheat oven to 350 degrees F.
2. Spray 13x9 pan with cooking spray.
3. Sprinkle Montreal seasoning over chicken breasts and cook in skillet until there's no pink.
4. Put cauliflower in dish, add 2 tbsp. water, cover with plastic wrap and cook in microwave for 4 minutes.
5. Sauté cooking oil and onions until clear. Add in squash and sauté until soft.
6. Cut chicken into cubes and add to casserole dish with vegetable. Pour Alfredo sauce over the top of dish.
7. Top with cheese and bread crumbs and bake for 20 minutes, and then boil for 10 until top of dish is brown.

Number of servings: 8

Macros (per serving):

Calories: 240.1
Protein: 26.9 g
Carbs: 6.9 g

Fat: 12.0 g

Scrambled Eggs

Ingredients:

- 1/4 cup green bell pepper, finely chopped
- 1 tbsp. onion, finely chopped
- 2 large eggs
- 1/4 cup low-fat cottage cheese
- 2 tbsp. low-fat cheddar cheese
- 2 tbsp. salsa

Directions:

1. Beat eggs and cottage cheese together.
2. Spray nonstick skillet with cooking spray.
3. Cook peppers and onions on medium heat until tender, roughly 2 minutes.
4. Add egg mixture and cheddar cheese.
5. Reduce heat to medium. Cook until set, stirring as needed.
6. Put the salsa on top and enjoy!

Number of servings: 1

Macros (per serving):

Calories: 274.8
Protein: 24.3 g
Carbs: 7.9 g
Fat: 14.5 g

Pork Chops for Crockpot

Ingredients:

- 10 pork chops
- 1 can low fat chicken cream soup
- 1/2 cup ketchup

Directions:

1. Put the pork chops into the crockpot.
2. Add in the soup and ketchup.
3. Cover the crockpot and cook on low for 8-9 hours.
4. Serve and enjoy!

Number of servings: 10

Macros (per serving):

Calories: 239.7
Protein: 21.8 g
Carbs: 8.2 g
Fat: 12.1 g

Cottage Cheese Breakfast

Ingredients:

- 1 cup 1% cottage cheese
- 1 tsp. ground cinnamon
- 1 packet Splenda
- 1/4 cup chopped almonds

Directions:

1. Put the cottage cheese, cinnamon, and Splenda in a bowl and mix well.
2. Sprinkle the chopped almonds on top and enjoy!

Number of servings: 1

Macros (per serving):

Calories: 249.8
Protein: 30.8 g
Carbs: 14.9 g
Fat: 8.6 g

Cheddar Bread

Ingredients:

- 1 large egg
- 2 tsp. flax seed meal
- 1/2 tbsp. baking powder
- 1 packet Splenda
- 1/4 cup shredded cheddar cheese
- 1 tsp. melted butter

Directions:

1. Melt butter in flat bowl or 15 oz. oval ramekin.
2. Add in the egg, flax meal, baking powder, Splenda, cheddar cheese and mix well.
3. Put in the microwave for 1 minute.
4. Flip over and cook for another 10 seconds until cooked throughout.
5. Cut in half, serve with favorite sandwich fillings and enjoy!

Number of servings: 1

Macros (per serving):

Calories: 289.2
Protein: 16.4 g
Carbs: 5.4 g
Fat: 22.5 g

Beef and Turkey Meatloaf

Ingredients:

- 3 1/2 lbs. ground turkey
- 3 1/2 lbs. ground beef
- 1 cup chopped onion
- 1 cup shredded carrots
- 1 sleeve saltine crackers
- 1/2 cup non-fat milk
- 4 large eggs
- 1 tbsp. salt
- 1 tbsp. pepper
- 2 tbsp. Worcestershire sauce
- 6 chopped cloves of garlic

Directions:

1. Preheat oven to 350 degrees F.
2. In a large bowl, crumble up the crackers and soak them in the milk for 15 minutes.
3. Chop the vegetables and add remaining ingredients to the cracker bowl.
4. Mix all of the ingredients in the bowl together until combined.
5. Form the combined mixture into a rectangle load in a 13x9 baking dish.
6. Bake for 80-90 minutes or until internal temp. reaches 160 degrees.
7. Cool for 10 minutes, serve, and enjoy!

Number of servings: 12

Macros (per serving):

Calories: 467.1
Protein: 21.7 g
Carbs: 8.5 g

Fat: 31.7 g

Taco Salad

Ingredients:

- 1 lb. extra lean ground beef
- 1 pkg. old El Paso taco seasoning
- 3/4 cup water
- 2 tbsp. olive oil
- 4 cups shredded romaine lettuce
- 1/2 cup chopped tomatoes
- 8 tbsp. fat free sour cream
- 1 cup shredded cheddar cheese

Directions:

1. Chop lettuce and set aside with tomatoes, cheese and sour cream.
2. Brown the beef with olive oil in skillet until thoroughly cooked.
3. Add in the taco seasoning and water to the skillet.
4. Simmer until water is reduced and remove from heat when done.
5. In 4 bowls, put one cup of lettuce in each bowl.
6. Add ¼ cup chopped tomatoes, beef, and cheese to each bowl.
7. Then add two tbsp. of sour cream to each bowl, serve and enjoy!

Number of servings: 4

Macros (per serving):

Calories: 489.0
Protein: 31.0 g
Carbs: 9.6 g
Fat: 36.1 g

Chile Casserole

Ingredients:

- 2- 7 oz. cans of green chilies
- 8 oz. shredded pepper-jack cheese
- 3 eggs
- 3/4 cup heavy cream
- 1/2 tsp. salt
- 4 oz. shredded cheddar cheese

Directions:

1. Grease an 8x8-baking pan and preheat oven to 350 degrees F.
2. Slice each chili along the long side and open to where it lays flat.
3. Arrange half of the chilies on one side of the pan, skin side down in a single layer.
4. Top the chilies with pepper-jack cheese.
5. Put the remaining chilies on top of the cheese, skin side up.
6. Beat the eggs, cream, and salt well, and then pour over the chilies.
7. Top with cheddar cheese and bake in oven for 35 minutes or until golden brown.
8. Let it cool off for 12 minutes, serve and enjoy!

Number of servings: 9

Macros (per serving):

Calories: 211.0
Protein: 10.9 g
Carbs: 1.4 g
Fat: 17.6 g

Chapter 10: Frequently Asked Questions

What if I'm not losing or gaining weight eating 13 calories per pound of bodyweight?

If you've been struggling to lose weight eating 13 calories per pound of bodyweight, then I recommend using a different method to set your calories. Before I get into that though, you must first make sure you were actually eating 13 calories per pound of bodyweight minus 500 calories to lose 1 pound per week. It's easy to overestimate the amount of calories you're eating, and this could be the reason why you're not seeing results.

Once you've made sure you've accurately been tracking your calories, you can take your goal bodyweight, multiply it by 11 and then eat that many calories (don't subtract anything from the final calculated number).

Yes, I understand that your goal bodyweight will be a random number that you think you'll look good at, so take your best guess. Start on the higher side and work your way down from there if you still aren't losing weight.

Here's an example for a 250-pound male.

Current Weight 250

Goal Bodyweight 200

200 x 11= 2,200 daily calories

Let's say once this person reaches his goal of 200 pounds, he's still not satisfied with how he looks. From there, he can simply set a new goal bodyweight (i.e. 190 pounds for example) and go from there.

On the other hand, let's say you're struggling to add muscle eating 13 calories per pound of bodyweight plus 250 calories. Again, make sure you're accurately tracking the amount of calories you're eating. You could be miscounting your calories, and that would account for why you're not gaining any weight. Once you've made sure you're tracking things accurately, you can add 100 calories to your total resting metabolic rate weekly until you start gaining weight. For example:

A 180-pound male looking to gain weight would multiply his bodyweight by 13 to determine his maintenance calories.

180 x 13= 2,340

This person would then add 250 calories to 2,340 and get a total of 2,590 calories per day. If he eats 2,590 calories on a daily basis, he should start to gain 0.5 pound per week. However, if he doesn't, he can simply add 100 calories to his original 2,590 calories on a weekly basis until he does.

For example, on week 1, he would eat 2,690 calories. If he didn't gain any weight by the end of the week, he would eat 2,790 calories for the following week, and so on and so forth until he starts gaining weight.

What if I hit a plateau and I stop losing weight at my regular pace?

Let's say you've been losing weight just fine, but then all of the sudden you hit a wall and stop losing weight. In this case, take your new current bodyweight (which should be a lower number from when you first started) and multiply that by 13.

Take that number and subtract 250 from it. This will be your new daily caloric intake for you to lose weight.

This will have you losing weight at a rate of approximately 0.5 pound per week. You may have previously been losing weight at a rate of 1 pound per week, but now you'll lose at a rate of 0.5 pound per week.

This is because I don't want you to drastically reduce your calories all of the sudden, and because if you've hit a plateau, you're likely very close to hitting your goal weight anyway.

What do I do once I reach my goal bodyweight?

Contrary to what you might be thinking, things aren't going to be that much different from what you've been doing to lose weight. You still need to do flexible dieting and continue eating in the same manner that you previously were. This means that you should still keep the same eating schedule and keep eating similar meals to the ones that you were eating to lose weight.

However, there's one difference between maintenance and creating a caloric deficit to lose weight. The difference is that you get to consume more calories! How many calories? Well, this is pretty easy to figure out as a matter of fact.

Step #1: Determine at what rate you were losing weight (i.e. 1 pound per week).

Step #2: Translate pounds lost per week into calories.
    0.5 pound lost per week= 250 calories
    1 pound lost per week= 500 calories
    1.5 pounds lost per week= 750 calories

2 pounds lost per week= 1,000 calories, etc.

Step #3: Add in those additional calories to what you were previously eating to maintain your new weight.

For example, let's say someone was losing weight at a rate of 1 pound per week by eating 1,850 calories per day. Once he hits his goal weight, he needs to eat 2,350 calories (1,850+500) per day to maintain his new weight.

How much weight should I lift during the workouts?

Lift as much weight as you possibly can for the given rep range. Initially, you won't know how much weight to use, so you'll have to take your best guess. For example, let's say you're doing bench press for 8 reps. You think you can lift around 150 pounds for that many reps, but on your first set, you easily complete 10 reps.

This means the weight is too light and you need to increase it for the next set. On the next set, you lift 165 pounds and struggle to complete the 8th rep. This is what you want to happen, and it means you've found a good weight to use. Once you can complete all 3 sets for 8 reps with 165 pounds, move up to 170 the next time you bench press. If you can't complete 8 reps for all 3 sets, stick with 165 until you can. Here's an example:

Workout 1: Bench Press with 165 pounds
Set 1: 8 reps
Set 2: 8 reps
Set 3: 7 reps

Because you only completed 7 reps on the last set, stick with 165 for the next workout.

Workout 2: Bench Press with 165 pounds
Set 1: 8 reps

Set 2: 8 reps
Set 3: 8 reps

Because you completed all 3 sets for 8 reps, move up to 170 on your next workout with bench press.

Note: It's better to use a weight that's too heavy and miss a rep or two than it is to use a weight that's too light and leave some reps in the tank. For example, it's better to do 170 pounds and only complete 6 reps instead of 8 as opposed to using 155 pounds and stopping at 8 reps even though you could've easily done more reps.

How Fast Should I Lose Weight?

The more weight you have to lose, the faster the rate at which you can lose the weight. For example, if you have 50+ pounds to lose, you can lose weight at a rate of 2 pounds or more per week. If you only have 5 pounds to lose, then lose weight at a rate of 0.5 pound per week.

For most people, losing 1 pound per week is the sweet spot. You'll be creating an average caloric deficit of 500 calories daily. At this pace, you'll be losing weight fairly quickly, and you won't be miserable all of the time from a complete lack of calories.

How much water should I drink on a daily basis?

Your body is made up of about 60% water, so it's important to consume water for several reasons. Drinking water regularly:

- Helps keep your joints and ligaments fluid, which can help prevent injury
- Helps control your caloric intake
- Flushes out toxins
- Improves skin quality

- Improves kidney function
- Improves your focus

Many people recommend that you should drink 1 gallon of water per day. This is a blanket answer that doesn't meet individual needs. This recommendation would have a 100-pound woman drinking the same amount of water as a 200-pound man. Absurd!

Other health experts advise drinking eight 8-ounce glasses (64 ounces total) of water a day. But again 64 ounces isn't going to be enough for most people. What should you do then? I don't keep track of my water intake—I go by how I feel and the color of my urine.

Your body's own thirst mechanism will be accurate in telling you if you need more water. If you feel thirsty, go drink some water. If not, you're probably ok. You can also use the color of your urine to judge how hydrated you are. If your urine is yellow, then you should drink more water. If it's clear then you should be good to go. This keeps things simple and it's one less thing you have to keep track of.

Are there any supplements that you recommend I take?

Most supplements are a complete waste of money. There's not a single supplement that's required in order for you to build muscle or burn fat. In fact, I advise for the first 6 weeks of your IIFYM diet that you don't take *any* supplements at all.

This is because I want you to see for yourself that it really is possible for you to get results without supplements. Your hard work and dedication matter way more than any pill or powder.

With that being said, there are a few supplements I recommend if you have the budget for them:

#1: Protein Powder:

You can't have a recommended list of supplements without protein powder on the list, right? Just kidding. But this has to be one of the most overhyped supplements of all time.

I think that the media does a really good job of making us believe that we must take protein powder to build muscle or take it to prevent muscle loss. I do think that protein powder can provide some benefits if *you need it.*

If you struggle to consistently hit your macros with protein then I would consider investing in a protein powder. Protein is necessary to help build and prevent the breakdown of muscle.

Therefore, ensuring that your muscle is spared is a good thing. However, don't go out of your way and eat more calories just for the sake of consuming more protein.

#2: Fish/Krill Oil

These oils are great sources of Omega-3 fatty acids. This is a good thing because most people consume too many Omega-6 fatty acids with foods like vegetable and canola oil.

Ideally, you want to be consuming a 1 to 1 ratio of Omega-3's to Omega-6's. Fish and krill oil can help you narrow the gap between the two types of fatty acids that you're consuming.

The main benefit from consuming these oils is that they act as an anti-inflammatory in your body. When you consume Omega-6's on the other hand, they act as an inflammatory.

That's why it's important to strike a balance with both of the fatty acids. The anti-inflammatory benefit is great because it can reduce your risk of developing heart disease or high blood pressure.

Finally, reducing inflammation can aid in muscle recovery. If you're going to invest in fish or krill oil, make sure that it's a very high-grade supplement.

The way that some of the lower quality oils are processed inhibits the absorption of them, which would make them completely useless. As for investing in fish or krill oil, taking either one is fine really.

Krill oil does contain the antioxidant astaxanthin (17), which helps with joint health, boosts cognitive function and helps promote a healthy cholesterol balance, while fish oil does not. However, I have noticed that krill oil can be harder to find, and it's typically more expensive so don't sweat not buying it.

#3: Digestive Enzymes

This is my favorite supplement of all time, and it's probably one of the most underrated supplements as well. If your body can't absorb the vitamins and nutrients that you're consuming then what's the point?

The sad fact of the matter is that when our foods get cooked, many of the enzymes get destroyed. Digestive enzymes will not only help to replenish those enzymes missed from cooked foods, but it will also help your body to better break down and utilize the nutrients that you're eating.

Also, if you ever suffer regularly from bloating, heartburn or have bad skin, give digestive enzymes a try and see if you notice a difference. Of course, it's important to note that these enzymes need to be high quality if you want them to be of any use.

Simply going to the local grocery store and purchasing a $10 bottle of enzymes isn't going to cut it. You must buy a high-quality enzyme if you want to get any use out of it. Personally, I recommend using Bio Trust.

How Do I Motivate Myself to Go to the Gym?

Finding the motivation to go to the gym or eat right can be hard. No matter who you are, there will be times when you don't feel like working out. Having that feeling is ok, but you can't let it control you. There will be times when you'll have to do it anyway even when you don't feel like it.

That's what will ultimately separate a long-term successful fitness journey from failing at it. I do have some tips to help you out along the way:

Tip #1: Focus on Gradual Improvements

Many people make fitness an all-or-nothing game. They tell themselves that they'll workout 5 days a week and eat clean 100% of the time for the rest of their lives. Let's say you workout only 4 days one week. Are you a failure?

Of course not! You still worked out 4 days, but in your mind you are because you failed to reach 5 workouts. You make it hard to celebrate any small successes that you do have because the standards are too high.

Instead, focus on making smaller, more gradual improvements and celebrate any successes you have along the way. For example, start off with a goal to only workout 2 days per week if it's been years since you've last worked out. Once you achieve that goal, you'll feel good about yourself then you can move up to working out 3 days per week and so on.

Tip #2: Action Leads Motivation

People think they have to get the inspiration or motivation from somewhere in order to take the action necessary to workout. The reverse of that is actually true. You need to start by taking an action no matter how small. And once you get started, you'll likely want to continue on with what you're doing.

When I think about everything I have to do to workout such as put my gym clothes on, drive to the gym, workout with a bunch of grueling exercises, drive back and shower, I start to make up silly excuses as to why I should skip this time. Instead, I'll tell myself to do just one exercise when I get to the gym and not pressure myself to do anything more. After I finish that first exercise, it's always easier for me to finish the rest of the workout.

You just have to get started. Try this out for any healthy habit you want to start. For example, if you want to start flossing your teeth, tell yourself you'll only floss one tooth and don't pressure yourself to do anything more than that!

Tip #3: Put Your Own Money on the Line

Money is a very powerful motivator. And you can use your own money to motivate yourself to start working out more. Here's what you're going to do—give someone a good amount of money. Not $20, but something that would actually hurt you—$100, $200, $500, or whatever you can't afford to lose.

Then tell your friend that if you don't go to the gym 3 days this week, for example, they get to keep the money. When you give up the money in the first place, you'll fight to get it back. This is much different than telling yourself you'll give the money to someone after you miss your workouts.

It's too easy to make an excuse and not give away the money. Give the money up in the first place and make sure your friend actually holds you accountable to it. This is by far the best way to get motivation to workout. There's a real cost involved if you don't comply. You'll either get ripped or go broke trying.

Conclusion

Thanks for getting this book and reading it all the way through to the end! The 5:2 diet is a good way to get and stay in shape for the rest of your life. You simply have to stay dedicated. The 5:2 diet will work as long as you put forth the effort needed.

Feel free to email me at thomas@rohmerfitness.com with any fitness questions you may have.

And finally, if this book was helpful, please take a few minutes and leave a review. Your feedback will help me make better content for you in the future!

Sources

(1)
https://www.ncbi.nlm.nih.gov/pubmed/22825659

(2)http://fitness.mercola.com/sites/fitness/archive
/2016/03/25/health-benefits-fasting.aspx#_edn1

(3) https://www.ncbi.nlm.nih.gov/pubmed/371355

(4)
https://www.ncbi.nlm.nih.gov/pmc/articles/PMC3
289210/

(5)
https://www.ncbi.nlm.nih.gov/pmc/articles/PMC3
289210/

(6)
https://www.ncbi.nlm.nih.gov/pmc/articles/PMC4
257368/

(7)
https://www.ncbi.nlm.nih.gov/pubmed/24993615

(8)
https://www.ncbi.nlm.nih.gov/pubmed/17929537

(9) http://www.mayoclinic.org/healthy-lifestyle/weight-loss/expert-answers/caffeine/faq-20058459

(10)
https://www.ncbi.nlm.nih.gov/pmc/articles/PMC4391809/

(11)
https://www.ncbi.nlm.nih.gov/pubmed/22460474

(12)
https://www.ncbi.nlm.nih.gov/pubmed/2796409

(13)
https://www.ncbi.nlm.nih.gov/pubmed/8028502

(14)
https://www.ncbi.nlm.nih.gov/pmc/articles/PMC1402378/

*Recipes inspired by users at sparkpeople.com